The UM-CIRHT Framework for Integrating Comprehensive Contraception and Abortion Care Competencies into Health Professions Education

Authors

Solomon W. Beza, MD, MPH, Bekalu M. Chekol, MA, Munir K. Eshetu, MD, Lia T. Gebremedhin, MD, MHA, Berhanu G. Gebremeskel, MD, MPH, Mengistu H. Damtew, MD

Contributors

Yolanda Smith, MD, MS, Alula Teklu, MD, MPH, Kathleen L. Omollo, SPP, MPP, MSI, Azeb T. Hailemeskel, MPH, MS, Janet Hall, MBA, Tamrat Endale, PhD, Daniel Rivkin, BA, Elizabeth Randolph, MSPH, Gurpreet K. Rana, MLIS

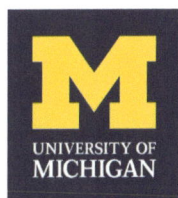

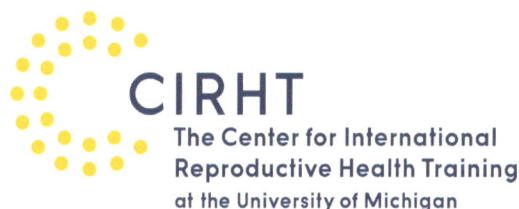

UNIVERSITY OF MICHIGAN

CIRHT
The Center for International
Reproductive Health Training
at the University of Michigan

UNIVERSITY OF MICHIGAN

CIRHT
The Center for International
Reproductive Health Training
at the University of Michigan

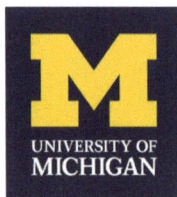

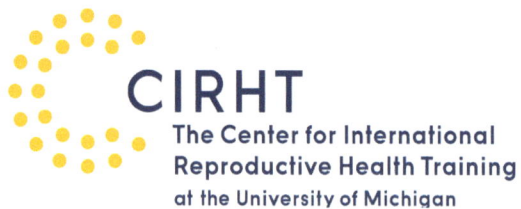

Published in the United States of America by
Michigan Publishing

ISBN 978-1-60785-513-2 (paper)

Contents

Acknowledgments

We wish to express our gratitude to Senait Fisseha, MD, JD, clinical adjunct professor of Obstetrics and Gynecology at the University of Michigan, the founder and first director of the Center for International Reproductive Health Training at the University of Michigan (UM-CIRHT). Her dedication to women and girls throughout the world is an inspiration to many. We are grateful to the University of Michigan and the faculty and leadership at our partner schools in Ethiopia and Rwanda. We extend our sincere thanks to all the trainees who are the beneficiaries of the training program in our partner schools.

We are appreciative of the Ministries of Health and Education of the Federal Democratic Republic of Ethiopia and the Ministry of Health in Rwanda for supporting the formal integration of family planning and comprehensive abortion care training into UM-CIRHT's partner medical and midwifery schools.

This framework document was made possible through a grant from an anonymous donor to UM-CIRHT.

The authors also gratefully acknowledge the editorial support of Michigan Publishing.

Acronyms

CAC	comprehensive abortion care
FP	family planning
FP/CAC	family planning and comprehensive abortion care
IUD	intrauterine device
LARC	long-acting reversible contraception
M&E	monitoring and evaluation
MVA	manual vacuum aspiration
Ob-Gyn	Obstetrics and Gynecology
OSCE	objective structured clinical examination
PPIUD	postpartum intrauterine device
PREPSS	Pre-Publication Support Service
QI	quality improvement
QoC	quality of care
RH	reproductive health
UM-CIRHT	Center for International Reproductive Health Training at the University of Michigan

Executive Summary

Each year, an estimated 73 million unintended pregnancies occur in the developing world, of which 49% end up in induced abortion with potential detrimental health and economic impact for women and their families.[1] Although there has been a marked reduction in unmet need for family planning across the globe over the last 25 years, the decline has been less pronounced in developing regions (16%) compared to developed world settings (30%).[2] One of the limitations in achieving substantial progress is inadequate access to trained professionals who are able to provide comprehensive reproductive health (RH) services, especially in contraception and comprehensive abortion care (CAC). Traditionally, preservice training in contraception and abortion in many developing countries was predominantly didactic, with limited hands-on training, so most medical and other midlevel health professionals graduated without the necessary competencies to provide these key RH services.

The underpinning of the framework developed by the Center for International Reproductive Health Training at the University of Michigan (UM-CIRHT) is the integration of competency-based training in contraception and CAC within curricula for medical, midwifery, and nursing students and Obstetrics and Gynecology (Ob-Gyn) residents. By exposing trainees to all competencies early on, students are expected to develop the requisite skills and values to provide comprehensive RH services after graduation, ultimately improving access and reducing morbidity and mortality from unintended pregnancy and unsafe abortion. To achieve this, UM-CIRHT partners with academic institutions to support curricular enhancement and ensure competency-based learning and assists in its implementation through various faculty development efforts and infrastructure enhancements, including simulation lab setup or augmentation.

Although UM-CIRHT's primary focus is training, the framework includes supporting institutions to develop model RH clinics that provide quality comprehensive clinical services in contraception and abortion. These clinics serve a dual purpose: They provide high-quality patient care that exemplifies compassion and respect for women and create a platform for practical training for midwifery, nursing, and medical students and Ob-Gyn residents in women-centered counseling, contraception, and CAC. They are designed to be easily accessible to all types of patients in the community, including those with disabilities, and they include all essential personnel, written standards of care, equipment, supplies, and pharmaceuticals. Continuous quality-improvement initiatives are integrated into the service provision to ensure access and quality of services with an emphasis on efficient, comprehensive, compassionate, and respectful care.

Although ample evidence demonstrates the impact of research in improving population health outcomes, there is a dearth of reproductive health research in most universities in developing nations. UM-CIRHT believes that findings from research can inform providers, policy makers, and the public and enhance the quality of training and eventually access and quality of care for women and girls. The foundation of UM-CIRHT's research support is identifying gaps in research practice and designing a comprehensive, tailored strategy to inculcate a research culture and build faculty capacity locally. With local and international trainers, UM-CIRHT conducts research methodology workshops at different milestones of the research continuum and provides ongoing mentorship to support the full cycle of the research process. This is enhanced by awarding seed grants that emphasize team science, supporting multidisciplinary research projects led by junior faculty investigators in Ob-Gyn, midwifery, and nursing departments.

In order to foster a thriving academic environment for education, clinical, and research programs, faculty development is integrated into these three core implementation arms. UM-CIRHT works with institutions and with local and international trainers on faculty development. Training is often conducted as workshops coupled with mentorship by the University of Michigan and other partners. Training topics depend on the need of each partner institution/country and usually include effective teaching and assessment, leadership, information resources literacy and evidence-based search strategies, research methodology, quality improvement, clinical skills in advanced contraception and abortion care, compassionate and respectful care, and counseling.

The goal of this framework document is to describe the approach UM-CIRHT uses to execute its core programmatic and operational strategies for interested countries and/or institutions that aspire to enhance preservice training in family planning and CAC in their particular settings.

Background

The Center for International Reproductive Health Training at the University of Michigan (UM-CIRHT) was founded with the mission of partnering with academic institutions in developing nations to strengthen their capacity to provide competency-based preservice training in family planning and comprehensive abortion care (FP/CAC). To achieve this, UM-CIRHT focuses on integrating competency-based training in FP/CAC into the various curricula, enhancing skills training, improving the quality of care in FP/CAC, and fostering a culture of research and building research capacity in reproductive health (RH).

The main goal is to enable partner institutions to graduate competent health professionals who are able to deliver high-quality, comprehensive RH services to women and girls, ultimately improving access and reducing morbidity and mortality from unintended pregnancy and unsafe abortion.

UM-CIRHT is a grant-funded center founded in 2014 by Senait Fisseha, MD, JD, who was its first executive director. The center was initially housed within the Department of Obstetrics and Gynecology at the University of Michigan until July 2017, when UM-CIRHT transitioned to an independent unit under the auspices of Michigan Medicine administration. UM-CIRHT's approach aligns with the three functions of academic medical institutions: education, clinical service, and research. UM-CIRHT began its program implementation in one institution in Ethiopia, which expanded to nine additional partner universities across the country. The next partnership initiative was with the University of Rwanda, and UM-CIRHT plans to continue expanding its portfolio to include partnerships with institutions in other countries in Africa, Asia, and Latin America.

Rationale

The high incidence of unsafe abortion and the unmet need for effective contraception result in unacceptably high levels of maternal mortality and morbidity in developing countries. Among other reasons, the dearth of health care workers trained with the requisite comprehensive contraception and abortion skills is a contributory factor to this challenge, with graduates leaving their health professional schools unprepared to provide RH services such as long-acting reversible contraceptive (LARC) placement and CAC.

Traditionally, countries have addressed the deficiency in RH service delivery through in-service competency training for a select number and mix of health professionals. Such supplemental stand-alone trainings, though important in increasing uptake of these services, are not sustainable and are likely less efficient and less cost-effective. Especially in the developing countries where there are few public service providers to address the diverse health care needs of a growing populace, an in-service training strategy may potentially aggravate the human resource crisis by diverting those same public health sector workers away from their patients during the time that they are training.

Teaching these critical skills to trainees while they are still in school through integration of content into the curriculum and utilization of a competency-based training method is a potentially more effective approach to overcome these challenges as demonstrated by our comparative study in Ethiopia.[3]

UM-CIRHT designed a framework that is aimed at ensuring acquisition of the needed competencies for provision of contraception and abortion care in a preservice education setting. This framework was adapted from the Ryan Residency Training Program, which strives to integrate and enhance abortion and contraception training for Ob-Gyn residents in the United States and Canada.[4]

Framework

The goal of UM-CIRHT's framework is to support the capacity-building of partner universities to graduate health care providers competent to deliver high-quality contraception and safe pregnancy termination services. Capacity-building includes:

- ensuring the formal integration of a comprehensive and competency-based curriculum in contraception and abortion across the different preservice training programs; and
- conducting tailored faculty development initiatives targeted at improving clinical, teaching, research skills to enable high-quality competency-based training in FP/CAC;
- ensuring the needed infrastructure is in place to achieve the successful implementation of the competency-based training with adequate opportunities for hands-on and simulation-based clinical training.

The UM-CIRHT framework targets all levels of health care providers but focuses on the preservice training of medical students, interns, Ob-Gyn residents, midwives, and nurses. The approach is aligned with the tripartite mission of academic medical centers: education and training, clinical service, and research, with faculty development embedded in all three core areas. The framework has been designed to align the strategies for each of those areas with the overall goal of training competent health care providers. It also reinforces the interconnectedness among education, service, and research to create graduates who have all the competencies required to provide comprehensive RH services.

UM-CIRHT's framework is grounded in the principles of mutual respect and authentic collaboration with partner institutions. A clear measure of success would be that the partner institution shows a commitment to implement and sustain the program beyond the end date of UM-CIRHT's direct support. To achieve this, UM-CIRHT ensures that the in-country partner institutions take ownership and are at the forefront, leading the program, with UM-CIRHT having a supportive role starting from the early phase of establishing collaborations. In addition, the sustainability plan is incorporated for each program beginning at the planning phase.

This framework is intended to provide guidance on how the programmatic and operational strategies for FP/CAC could be executed in other countries or institutions that seek to replicate the UM-CIRHT model in their settings. The framework may be adapted to the local context of individual countries and institutions. This document is divided into two sections: the programmatic dimensions of the framework and the operational dimension for effective implementation as a program.

SECTION 1
Programmatic Dimensions of the Framework

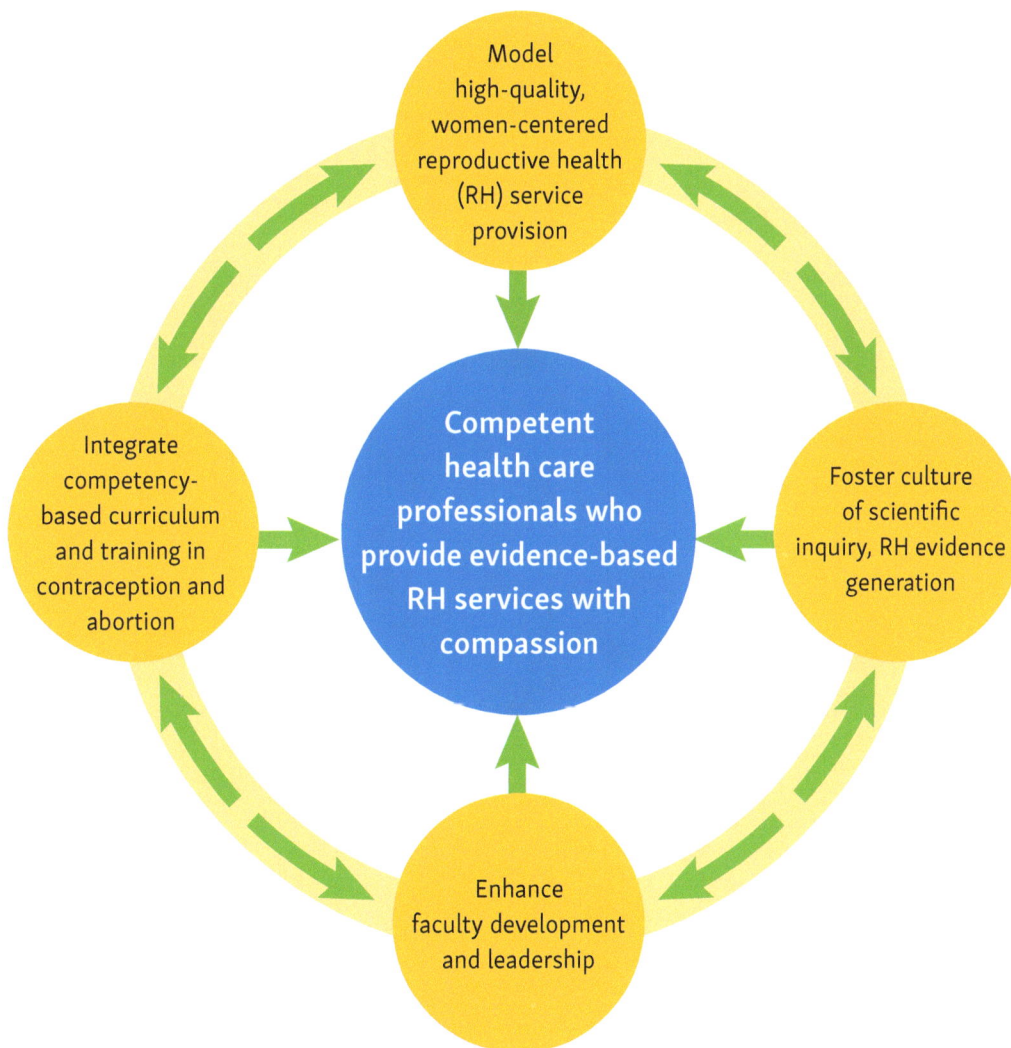

Figure 1. Relationship among core strategic areas

1.1 Strategies for Education

To enhance training on contraception and comprehensive abortion care (CAC) skills (Figure 1) the Center for International Reproductive Health Training at the University of Michigan (UM-CIRHT) works with partners to address the whole continuum of curriculum, beginning with reviewing the curriculum, modifying it as needed into competency-based training, and monitoring and evaluating the implementation (Figure 2). The partner institution (and, where applicable, the local ministry of health and/or ministry of education) leads the review and revision process, which serves as a gateway to the critical changes aimed at creating and sustaining the envisioned competency-based program.

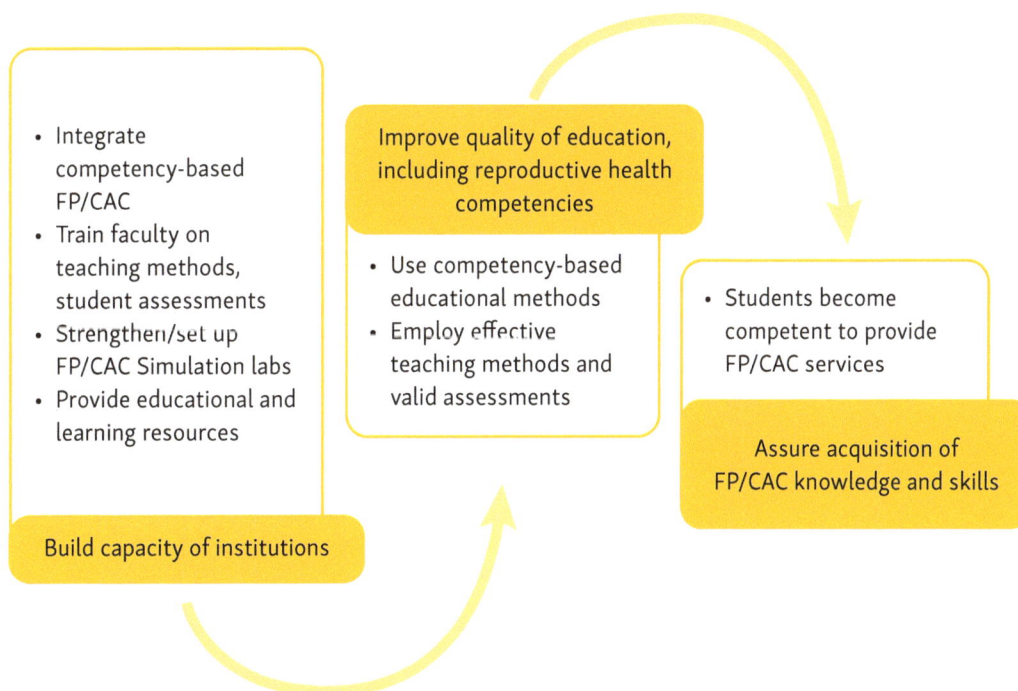

- Integrate competency-based FP/CAC
- Train faculty on teaching methods, student assessments
- Strengthen/set up FP/CAC Simulation labs
- Provide educational and learning resources

Build capacity of institutions

Improve quality of education, including reproductive health competencies

- Use competency-based educational methods
- Employ effective teaching methods and valid assessments

- Students become competent to provide FP/CAC services

Assure acquisition of FP/CAC knowledge and skills

Figure 2. Strategies to build capacity with institutions to enhance reproductive health education

Review and Revise the Curriculum

To be able to promote the acquisition of specific competencies, they must be clearly outlined in the written curriculum. UM-CIRHT supports the revision of curriculum so that provision of family planning and comprehensive abortion care (FP/CAC) services is formally incorporated into the overall training curriculum of the schools. The curriculum must include detailed course syllabi that outline learning outcomes and align with teaching methods and assessments.

Implement Revised Curriculum

A well-written curriculum by itself does not guarantee its delivery unless there is faculty engagement and availability of teaching and learning resources. After leadership endorses the curriculum, faculty are oriented on the revision and provided a series of on-site workshops on effective teaching focusing on skills-teaching and case-based learning (Appendix 1). Educational resources, such as voice-over PowerPoint presentations, case studies, and videos for skills demonstration to standardize delivery of content, are developed in collaboration with faculty in partner institutions.

Faculty are expected to direct students to acquire the skills in a safe and simulated environment before they are given the opportunity to practice on patients. This improves their confidence, providing ample opportunities to make and learn from mistakes. In addition, this strategy ensures patient safety. Promoting skills-teaching in simulated settings and setting up or enhancing skill/simulation labs with necessary equipment, including pelvic and arm models and other simulators, need to be backed by advocacy for simulation teaching. These are key aspects of UM-CIRHT's support. For the appropriate management and maintenance of the clinical skills / simulation labs, individuals are trained to oversee the labs, facilitate sessions, coordinate schedules, handle equipment, and manage sim labs. The other key component of the hands-on training is incorporating dedicated rotations of trainees in FP clinics. During these rotations, use of logbooks is emphasized to reinforce students' learning on skills at clinical sites.

Robust assessment methods are the best way to ensure quality of education and drive continuous learning. Faculty are trained in writing context-dependent item sets that test students' abilities to apply concepts and principles rather than merely recall facts. They are also trained on how to design and run objective structured clinical examination (OSCE) stations to objectively assess students' clinical decision-making, communication, and psychomotor skills objectively. Partner schools are supported to have exam blueprints and exam banks. UM-CIRHT's technical team provides on-site mentorship and feedback during actual teaching, test question development, and OSCE station setup whenever feasible.

Cultivate Leadership Among Faculty

All faculty have some level of leadership requirements. For department chairs or directors who oversee teaching, mentoring, and supervising, the responsibilities are more pronounced. Faculty at all levels require leadership competencies to effectively implement and communicate change, take proactive roles in their departments, be self-aware and reflective, use problem-solving and decision-making skills, be strong role models, and inspire their students. UM-CIRHT's model incorporates faculty development in educational leadership that includes periodic workshops complemented by regular mentoring and coaching (Figure 3).

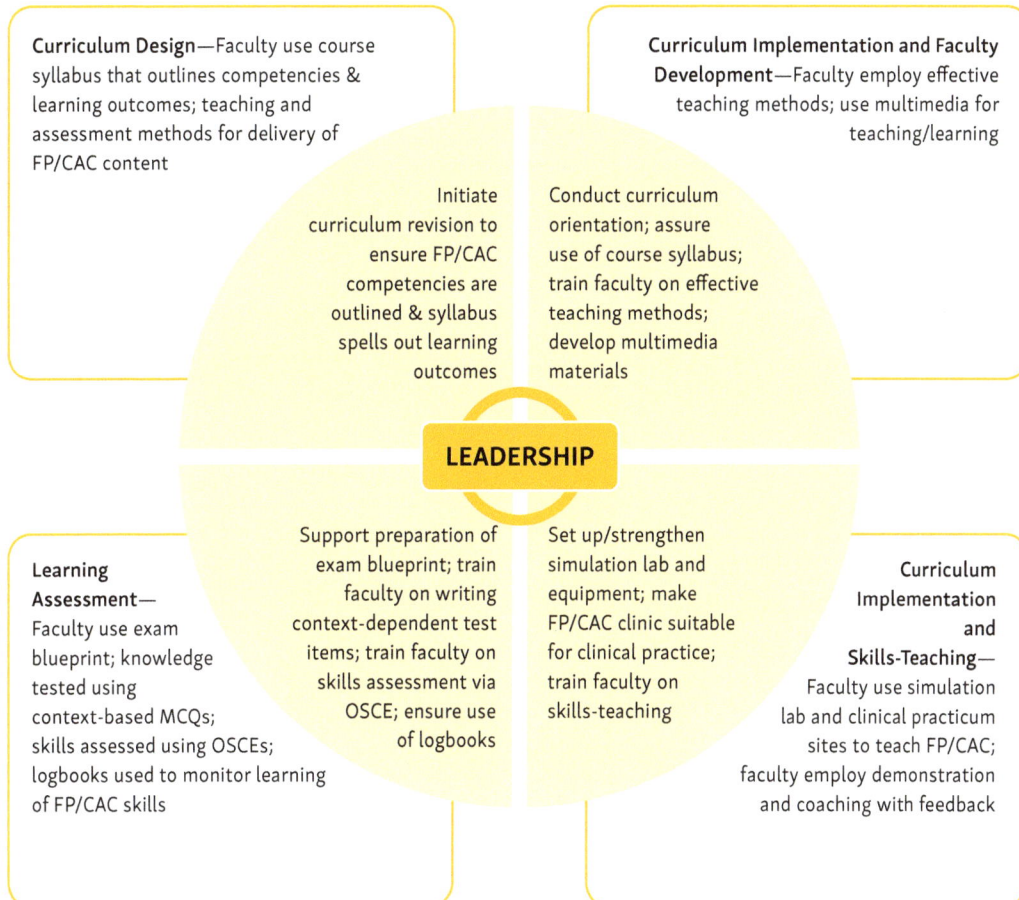

Curriculum Design—Faculty use course syllabus that outlines competencies & learning outcomes; teaching and assessment methods for delivery of FP/CAC content

Initiate curriculum revision to ensure FP/CAC competencies are outlined & syllabus spells out learning outcomes

Curriculum Implementation and Faculty Development—Faculty employ effective teaching methods; use multimedia for teaching/learning

Conduct curriculum orientation; assure use of course syllabus; train faculty on effective teaching methods; develop multimedia materials

LEADERSHIP

Learning Assessment—Faculty use exam blueprint; knowledge tested using context-based MCQs; skills assessed using OSCEs; logbooks used to monitor learning of FP/CAC skills

Support preparation of exam blueprint; train faculty on writing context-dependent test items; train faculty on skills assessment via OSCE; ensure use of logbooks

Set up/strengthen simulation lab and equipment; make FP/CAC clinic suitable for clinical practice; train faculty on skills-teaching

Curriculum Implementation and Skills-Teaching—Faculty use simulation lab and clinical practicum sites to teach FP/CAC; faculty employ demonstration and coaching with feedback

Figure 3. Model to ensure competency on contraception and comprehensive abortion care (CAC) training

1.2 Strategies for Clinical Service

Teaching and referral hospitals in developing countries generally give less emphasis to the delivery of contraception and abortion care services and often relegate these services to lower-level facilities such as primary hospitals or community health centers. Hence less emphasis is given to the physical infrastructure and/or the overall quality and comprehensiveness of these services. This is a missed opportunity for women to access RH care at referral hospitals, as there is a high volume of patients coming for other medical, surgical, or Ob-Gyn care. This also minimizes the exposure of all trainees for hands-on practice of contraception and abortion in teaching hospitals.

The Center for International Reproductive Health Training (UM-CIRHT) framework focuses on establishing clinics that model a women-friendly, compassionate, and respectful health care environment. By training in those facilities, students are encouraged to become champion providers and observe and contribute to the quality of care being delivered. A robust service with a high patient volume increases opportunities for hands-on practice, thus enhancing trainees' skills. The aim is to enable students to become competent and compassionate providers and advocates for these services (Figure 4). The framework incorporates the improvement of the quality and utilization of contraception and abortion services using the following interventions.

Establish a Model Clinic for Contraception and Safe Abortion

Identifying and appropriating adequate, dedicated space to serve as a model clinic that is women-friendly is an important step in strengthening contraception and abortion services in teaching hospitals. The model clinic provides comprehensive abortion and contraceptive services and related reproductive health (RH) services, including care for victims of sexual assault and adolescent RH services. The model clinic is easily accessible to all types of patients, including those with disabilities, and includes all the essential equipment, supplies, and drugs needed to provide contraception and abortion care. The clinic must have an adequate number of providers who are competent in the provision of women- and

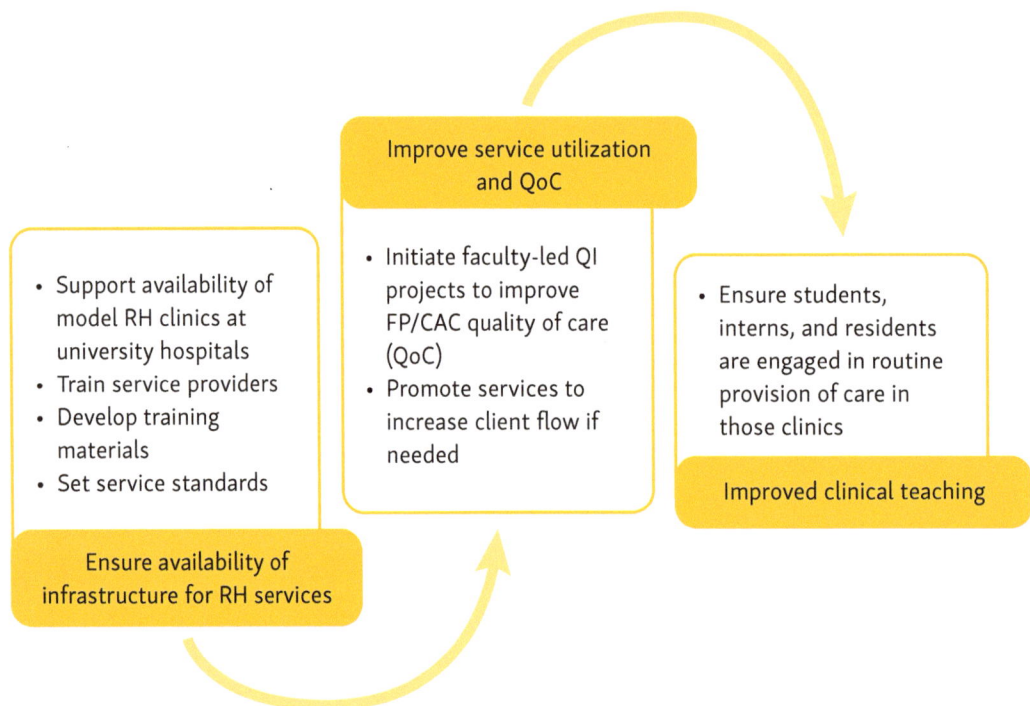

Improve service utilization and QoC

- Initiate faculty-led QI projects to improve FP/CAC quality of care (QoC)
- Promote services to increase client flow if needed

- Support availability of model RH clinics at university hospitals
- Train service providers
- Develop training materials
- Set service standards

Ensure availability of infrastructure for RH services

- Ensure students, interns, and residents are engaged in routine provision of care in those clinics

Improved clinical teaching

Figure 4. Strategies to improve reproductive health clinical services with institutions

adolescent-friendly contraception and abortion services and must include written standards of care for all services. Depending on the existing infrastructure and needs of each partner institution, UM-CIRHT's support may range from making simple renovations to constructing a new facility (usually with matching institutional funds), equipping the model clinic, and training the institutions' staff. Training for the clinic physicians, nurses, and other staff ranges from knowledge and skills in family planning and comprehensive abortion care (FP/CAC) to compassionate care, counseling, and professionalism.

Initiate and Sustain Quality Improvement Projects

An important aspect of engaging faculty in contraception and abortion care is involving them in initiatives to improve the quality of care. Initiating quality improvement (QI) projects that are designed and implemented by designated QI teams composed of nurses, midwives, residents, and faculty has multiple benefits. First and foremost, the projects can directly improve quality of care and client satisfaction, leading to increased client numbers. They can also maximize students' opportunity to practice in a high-quality service environment, affording the opportunity to inspire these future professionals to replicate such services in their respective facilities following graduation. They introduce them to the concept that QI is a never-ending process throughout their careers. The lessons learned in improving the quality of contraception and abortion services can also have a spillover effect in improving the quality of care of other medical services.

The QI projects begin by assessing the quality of care against a set of standards and identifying potentially innovative improvement ideas, which may also include the goal of increasing utilization of services. QI committees then meet regularly to assess the progress and implementation of the interventions. Outcomes of the projects will be published to disseminate the experience gained and encourage and motivate faculty and staff. The service improvements and resulting best practices outcomes may also be shared in national and international forums.

Engage Medical and Midwifery Students, Interns, and Ob-Gyn Residents in the Routine Provision of Reproductive Health Care

Once a dedicated contraception and abortion service with good client volume is established, students, interns, and residents are involved in the provision of routine care as part of their practical training. Final-year midwifery students, interns, and Ob-Gyn residents are assigned to the model clinic and are encouraged to be involved in the QI projects and in the collection, interpretation, and presentation of clinical service data to the department. The staff in the model clinic are also trained on how to supervise students during service provision.

1.3 Strategies for Research

Findings from reproductive health (RH) research can provide vital information that will inform health policy, reinforce efforts to protect women's and adolescents' access to quality health care, and improve population health outcomes. However, there is a paucity of RH research output from most universities in developing nations due in part to a lack of knowledge and skills in research conduct, time constraints, and limited or no funding. This is usually compounded by institutional structure that is not conducive to scientific inquiry.

Fostering a Research Culture

Fostering research culture begins with assessing the status of research practices and the factors affecting research activities at the partner institution to inform best strategies. Based on those findings, a comprehensive research strategy is codesigned and tailored to each institution's need (Figure 5).

Seasoned clinician investigators are invited to share lessons on conducting research amid busy clinical schedules. The purpose of these inspirational talks is to inspire young investigators and demystify the research endeavor. Following a workshop on framing research questions, competitive seed grants are awarded through a call for concept notes and specific aims for research in RH with a focus on family planning and comprehensive abortion care (FP/CAC). The selection of research projects is based on set criteria.

Building Research Capacity

To inculcate a research culture and build research capacity, the following framework is employed:

- A platform is created to enhance the quality of research protocol development through hands-on workshops.
- Competitive research grants are awarded following ranking by expert research reviewers and may include input from the partner's ministry of health.
- A series of training workshops is conducted across the continuum of the research cycle, from developing the research question(s) to publishing the results. Milestones include the following:
  - framing a research question
  - developing research protocol (encouraging team science)
  - managing research
  - collecting and analyzing data
  - manuscript writing
  - selecting and submitting to peer-reviewed journals and conferences

- The workshops are delivered as hands-on trainings and are tailored, phase-based, and conducted on-site whenever feasible.
- Mentorship is provided through pairing with faculty at the University of Michigan or other institutions with relevant expertise.
- Pre-Publication Support Service at the University of Michigan provides faculty peer review and writing support to help improve manuscripts for competitive submissions for publication in peer-reviewed academic journals (https://sites.google.com/umich.edu/prepss).

The overall approach builds on ideas from social cognitive theory, including focusing on modeling positive behavior and improving self-efficacy and social persuasion.

Key Principles of a Research Program

- **On-Site Training:** Since removing faculty and other health care providers from their respective workstations creates service interruptions, research-related trainings are done on-site whenever possible. The schedule is arranged with consideration of faculty convenience to minimize any disruptions to service and/or teaching.
- **Team Science:** The research teams must have at least four members to be eligible for research support/grants. Quality improvement (QI) projects must also have a multidisciplinary team of health care providers.
- **Learning:** Each step in the research cycle is viewed as a learning opportunity.

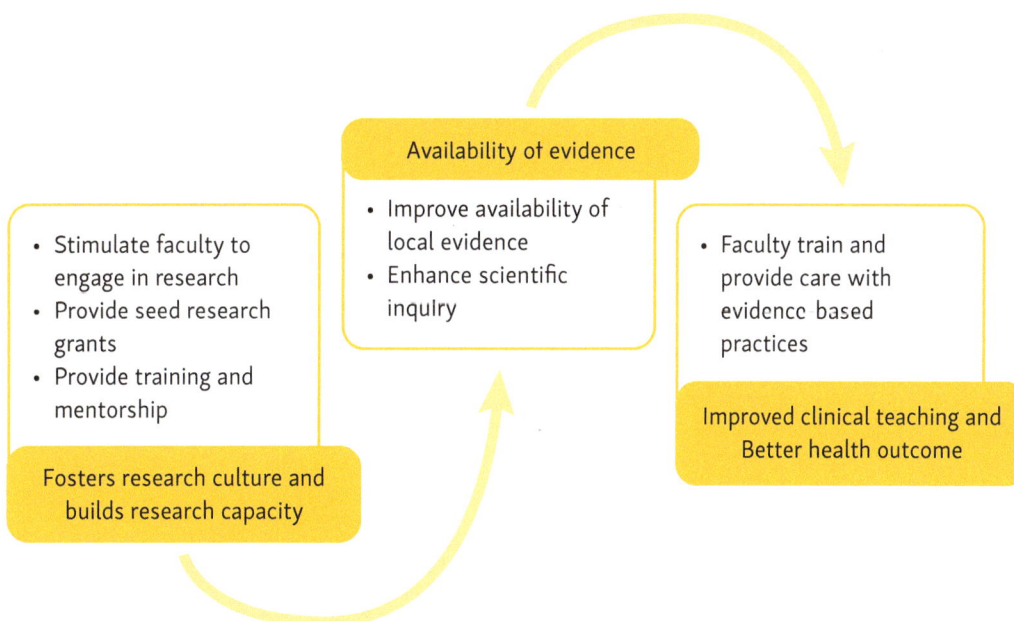

Availability of evidence

- Improve availability of local evidence
- Enhance scientific inquiry

- Stimulate faculty to engage in research
- Provide seed research grants
- Provide training and mentorship

Fosters research culture and builds research capacity

- Faculty train and provide care with evidence based practices

Improved clinical teaching and Better health outcome

Figure 5. Strategies to improve faculty research that aims to enhance reproductive health service and teaching

- **Workforce Development:** Faculty who have research skills are identified to co-facilitate research training for the same institution. If an external trainer is needed, training is designed with the goal to create a local pool of trainers who can be tapped for future cascading of the training education of other faculty and trainees.
- **Mentorship:** A strong mentorship program is developed for faculty, matching them with collaborators at their own or partner institutions. This relationship provides both additional research and career development support.
- **Tailored Support:** Customized support is provided to each team based on their needs and their pace. When one research team makes progress and advances in the research cycle, support is given to maintain momentum. Data analysis support is also individualized to the research methodology and data needs of each team.

Collaborative Research Grants

The Center for International Reproductive Health Training (UM-CIRHT) also has a program through which competitive grants are awarded to collaborative research projects between faculty at the University of Michigan and faculty in UM-CIRHT partner countries. These grants are awarded to partner faculty who already have basic research skills. In addition to funding the selected projects, these teams are also supported through more advanced research training on relevant areas identified in their proposals.

SECTION 2
Operational Dimension of the Framework

For program implementation, the Center for International Reproductive Health Training at the University of Michigan (UM-CIRHT) collaborates primarily with universities in developing countries that have health science training programs in medicine, nursing, and midwifery. Based on each country's need, UM-CIRHT also works closely with respective ministries of health and/or education, although the direct partnership is primarily with colleges and universities. Partnerships may be initiated by UM-CIRHT, the partner institution, or the national ministry of health. Once a decision is made to launch a partnership with a university, a situational analysis is conducted by UM-CIRHT followed by collaborative planning based on the results of these findings and identified needs. The funding mechanism for expenses that will be incurred in-country is executed through a subcontract that UM-CIRHT coordinates with the partner university through the University of Michigan.

Although the program is supported by UM-CIRHT, it is fully owned by the partner institutions during implementation and after project completion. To run the in-country implementation, UM-CIRHT's core team works with in-country staff and the faculty at the partner universities. The core UM-CIRHT team and the in-country staff provide administrative and technical support to the institutional faculty who lead the implementation. One of the core principles of the UM-CIRHT model is to design and implement a program that can be sustained by the partner institution without creating the need for long-term external funding or support. From the beginning of the implementation process, an understanding of the exit strategy is essential for all parties.

Monitoring and Evaluation

A monitoring and evaluation (M&E) strategy that generates evidence that adheres to site practicalities is crucial to continually improve program performance. The M&E strategies within the framework have been designed to provide needed project information; to enable effective, timely, systematic measurement of results for preparation of periodic reports; and to allow analysis of the reasons targets are or are not being achieved. The strategies detail the various types and sources of data that will be collected and used to evaluate measurable indicators.

The M&E strategy includes a range of indicators at various levels to measure, monitor, and evaluate both the implementation process and the outcomes of the Center for International Reproductive Health Training (UM-CIRHT) partnership. This strategy is based primarily on the logical framework approach and proposes that achieving specific results at different levels will lead to the desired impact (Figure 6). It combines the traditional logic model to depict the relationship between inputs, activities and outputs, outcomes, and impact with key strategies.

The M&E strategy focuses on the following objectives:

1. Identifying core indicators at various levels used to measure performance
2. Standardizing and streamlining data collection and reporting
3. Monitoring progress toward achieving outcomes
4. Evaluating how well the project has met the expected outcomes
5. Facilitating and promoting data utilization for informed decision-making

To collect the needed data for monitoring the program, institutions are supported to optimize the use of available data with their existing platforms without creating the need for any parallel systems. Using monthly reporting formats, data are collected by program site coordinators and compiled semiannually. To enhance the use of data to inform practice, supportive supervision is conducted at least quarterly, coupled with mentorship. All best practices are documented, reviewed, and made available for use by others and for publications.

Inputs

- University of Michigan faculty and staff trainers/mentors
- Regional local trainers
- UM-CIRHT staff
- Grant funding
- Dedicated research grant
- In-country partner school faculty and leadership
- Students/trainees
- Equipment
- Learning/educational resources
- Clinical/teaching
- Institutional guidelines/policies

Processes

- Create competency-based family planning and comprehensive abortion care (FP/CAC) curricula
- Develop faculty's clinical, teaching, and leadership skills in FP/CAC
- Improve skills/simulation labs for FP/CAC
- Strengthen FP/CAC clinics
- Establish multidisciplinary quality improvement (QI) teams/committees
- Train staff and faculty on compassionate and client-centered care
- Develop FP/CAC service standards and guidelines
- Provide research skills training and mentorship
- Provide research seed grants for faculty

Outputs

- Institutions with competency-based curriculum and detailed core syllabi in FP/CAC
- Faculty trained in clinical, teaching, and leadership skills in FP/CAC
- Fully functional simulation labs
- Dedicated FP/CAC clinics
- QI projects designed and implemented for FP/CAC services
- RH research projects designed by in-country research teams

Short-term outcomes

- Students engaged in FP/CAC hands-on practice
- Faculty provide competency-based training in FP/CAC
- Simulation-based training integrated into standard training
- RH clinics provide compassionate, integrated, and comprehensive FP/CAC services
- Increased number of clients receiving FP/CAC counseling and services in teaching hospital
- Improved client satisfaction
- Increased publications and presentations in RH research

Long-term outcomes

- Improved competence of students and residents in FP/CAC
- Strong institutional capacity for quality hands-on training in FP/CAC
- Quality, women-centered, accessible, comprehensive RH services
- Increased long-acting reversible contraceptive (LARC) use
- Increased number of faculty independent investigators
- Enhanced pool of locally available scientific evidence

Impact

- Reduced unintended pregnancies
- Reduced maternal morbidity and mortality from unintended pregnancies and unsafe abortions
- Critical mass of health professionals providing and advocating for RH services
- Culture of compassionate, respectful, women-centered care fostered
- Robust, self-sustaining institutional research culture

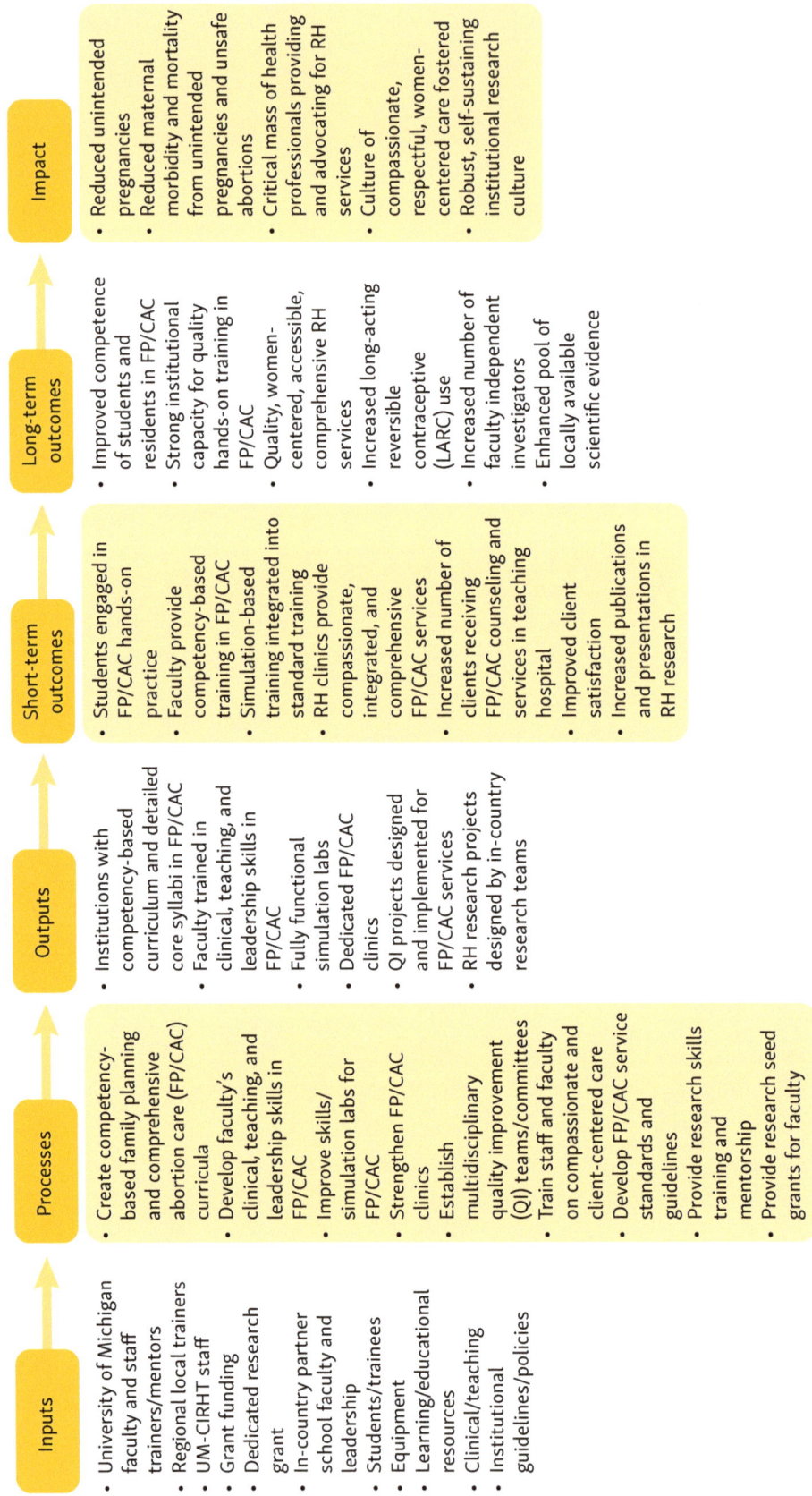

Figure 6. Monitoring and evaluation framework

References

1. Bongaarts, J., & Hardee, K. (2017, June). The role of public-sector family planning programs in meeting the demand for contraception in sub-Saharan Africa. *International Perspectives on Sexual and Reproductive Health, 43*(2), 41–50.

2. Bearak, J., Popinchalk, A., Alkema, L., & Sedgh, G. (2018). Global, regional, and sub-regional trends in unintended pregnancy and its outcomes from 1990 to 2014: Estimates from a Bayesian hierarchical model. *Lancet Global Health, 6*(4), e380–e389.

3. Gebremeskel B.G., Teklu A.M., Gebremedhin L.T., et al. (2018). Structured integration of family planning curriculum: Comparative assessment of knowledge and skills among new medical graduates in Ethiopia. *Contraception 98*, 89–94 DOI: 10.1016/j.contraception.2018.04.001

4. Steinauer, J.E., Turk, J.K., Fulton, M.C., Simonson, K.H., & Landy, U. (2013). The benefits of family planning training: A 10-year review of the Ryan Residency Training Program. *Contraception, 88*(2), 275–280.

Appendix 1

SAMPLE FAMILY PLANNING AND COMPREHENSIVE ABORTION CARE TOPICS IN VARIOUS CURRICULA

Topic
Didactics
1. Introduction to Family Planning and Abortion: Epidemiology
2. Medical Eligibility Criteria for Contraceptive Use
3. Counseling in Abortion and Family Planning
4. Short-term Contraceptives
5. Long-Acting Reversible Contraceptives (LARCs)
6. Permanent Methods of Contraception
7. Safe Abortion
8. Postabortion Care
9. Management of Abortion Complications
Simulation-Based Practice
10. Manual Vacuum Aspiration (MVA)
11. Interval IUD and PPIUD Insertion and Removal
12. Implant Insertion and Removal
13. Nonscalpel Vasectomy (Ob-Gyn Residents)
14. Bilateral Tubal Ligation (Ob-Gyn Residents)
15. Dilatation and Evacuation (Ob-Gyn Residents)
16. Laparoscopic Tubal Ligation (Ob-Gyn Residents)

Case-Based Discussions / Role Plays

17. Counseling

18. Professionalism, Value Clarification, and Empathy in Abortion Care: Legal and Ethical Dilemmas and Social Determinants

19. Medical Eligibility for Contraception

20. First-Trimester Bleeding

21. Care for Victims of Sexual Assault (Ob-Gyn Residents)

22. Medical and Surgical Abortion

23. Difficult Implant Removal (Ob-Gyn Residents)

Appendix 2

SAMPLE FACULTY DEVELOPMENT WORKSHOP/SEMINAR TOPICS

Topic

Education

1. Adult Learning Theory

2. How to Give an Interactive and Effective Presentation

3. Case-Based/Problem-Based Learning

4. How to Teach Using Simulation

5. Knowledge Assessment: Constructing Items That Test Application of Knowledge

6. Skills Assessment: How to Set Up and Conduct Objective Structured Clinical Examination (OSCE)

7. How to Give and Get Effective Feedback

8. Using Multimedia and Technology to Enhance Learning

9. Flipped Classroom Teaching

10. Peer-Assisted Learning

Clinical

11. Laparoscopic Tubal Ligations

12. Immediate Postpartum IUD

13. Dilatation and Evacuation

14. Obstetric Ultrasound

15. Pain Management

(continued)

SAMPLE FACULTY DEVELOPMENT WORKSHOP/SEMINAR TOPICS (*CONTINUED*)

Topic
Clinical
16. No Scalpel Vasectomy
17. Difficult Implant Removal
18. Value Clarification and Attitude Transformation: Empathy and Professionalism in Abortion Care
19. Patient-Centered Care
20. Designing and Implementing Quality Improvement (QI) Projects
Research
21. Framing a Research Question
22. Conducting Literature Search
23. Research Ethics
24. Overview of Study Designs and Research Methodology
25. Developing Research Protocol
26. Developing Data-Collection Instruments
27. Citation Management
28. Data Management
29. Data Analysis
30. Scientific Writing and Publishing
31. Grant Writing
32. Systematic Review and Meta-analysis
Leadership
33. Fundamentals of Leadership
34. Educational Leadership in Action
35. Becoming a Successful Mentor/Mentee

www.ingramcontent.com/pod-product-compliance
Lightning Source LLC
Chambersburg PA
CBHW042050210326
41520CB00044B/214